Controlling Panic

David Leahy

ISBN-13: 978-0995663022

ISBN-10:0995663025

Contents

1. Introduction - Why write this book

This is what I would have liked to have read when I was having the worst of my panic attacks. The only books I seen at the time (and still see now) are written by Doctors and Psychologists detailing the scientific basis of panic attacks, quoting studies for and against this and that theory, and offering no practical help to me in the midst of my suffering. If any did offer any treatment plan, it basically concentrated on treating the symptoms and not the disease, which is fine in the short term, but not really a viable long term solution – after all, life is long term (we hope!) Instead I hope to show the reader what I went through, and describe the hell, the frustration, the denial, the failed treatments and successful ones, and hope that the reader, if they are in any way suffering from any degree of anxiety disorder can benefit in some way from my experience. I'm not going to tell you what to do, I'm just going to describe what happened to me and hope that you can pick and choose some of the lessons that I learned and apply them to your own situation / condition. Because I know the awful hell of anxiety / panic attacks, if I can in any way help your condition, then it has been worth writing this book!

In short this book attempts to tell you:

- **What** is happening to you
- **Why** it's happening to you
- **How** to identify the causes and treat it

2. What is Panic?

When I check the oxford English dictionary for 'Panic' I get:

Panic
   • *noun 1 sudden uncontrollable fear or anxiety. 2 informal frenzied hurry to do something.* • *verb (panicked, panicking) feel or cause to feel panic. DERIVATIVES panicky adjective. — ORIGIN from the name of the Greek god Pan, noted for causing terror.*

I think the Greeks knew all about Panic Attacks, if they originated it from the Greek God for Terror!

And when I check the word 'Panic Attack' we get:

Panic Attack:
   • *noun a sudden overwhelming feeling of acute and disabling anxiety.*

The trouble is that these are just words, and up until you actually 'experience' a panic attack, you think of 'Panic' as something you do when you're going to miss your bus or lose your keys, and 'Anxiety' as something you might feel before an important test or exam. That's only natural, because we can only relate to the world in terms of our own experiences. I think a key word in this definition is 'disabling', because a panic attack can stop you in your tracks, or even prevent you from even venturing out of your house. When you 'panic' because you're going to miss your bus or lose your keys, it lasts at most a couple of minutes, and certainly doesn't 'disable you.

Anyone who has experienced a full blown panic or anxiety attack knows that it's nothing like losing your keys – it's 100 times worse. You think you're losing your mind – it's terrifying and reduces many sufferers to tears for no obvious reason.

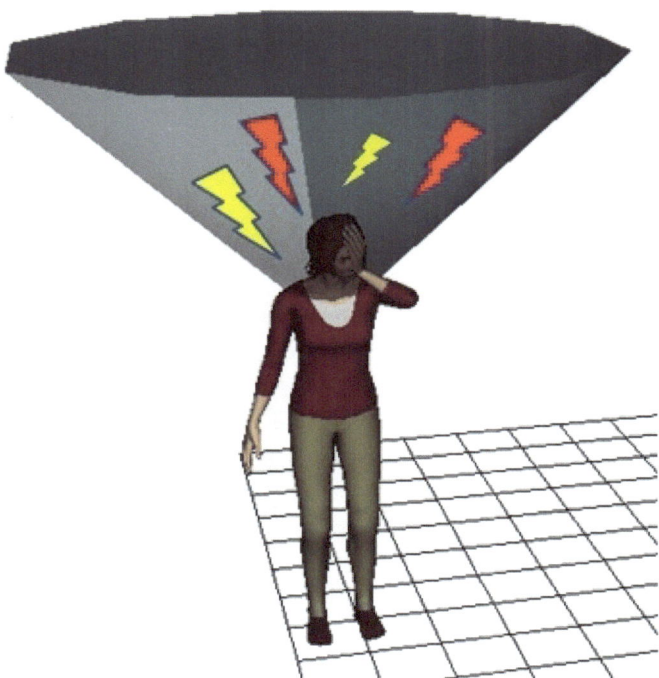

Figure 1 Visualization of Typical Panic Attack!

Panic is Good!

The truth is that panic is actually as good thing and has helped us and our ancestors to survive, as it is part of the fight-or-flight mechanism which helped us to avoid our natural predators (including other hostile humans) and live to fight another day. In this way 'panic' has evolved to help us, and still does in our modern environment, for example fearing fast moving cars when we're crossing the road, or fearing a long drop from a cliff edge. This is natural and helpful to help us to survive.

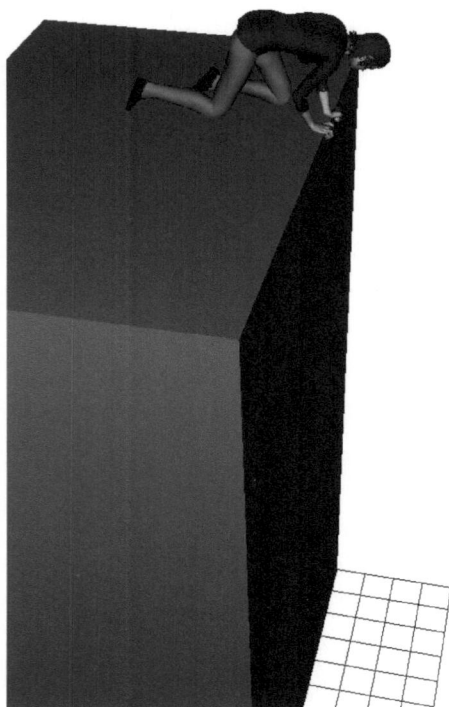

Figure 2 some panic is Good!

When I was studying Psychology in university we often referred to anxiety disorders etc. and we thought of anxiety as only something a bit stronger than we would feel just before an examination – it just shows how little we knew at the time.

A fully fledged panic attack is a very different animal indeed. It can come from nowhere – this awful indescribable feeling in your head of impending doom and that you are losing your mind, that something has gone wrong with the wiring in your brain and you are basically about to die! Other symptoms I personally have experienced are:

- Intense feeling of dread – like a heavy weight squeezing my brain
- Feeling that your head will explode
- Palpitations, sweating
- Confusion
- Thought patterns gone wrong
- Scalp tingling
- Throbbing blood vessels in your scalp
- Claustrophobic & agoraphobic
- Paranoia – everyone around me knows my head is about to explode
- Shivers and hot flushes
- Inability to concentrate on anything

I could go on – the list is endless. I'm told by the psychologists that it's the parasympathetic nervous system (normally put to good use to run from a lion) however in the middle of the street, or sitting at your office desks there are NO lions – in fact it would help if there were !

The unfortunate aspect to a typical panic attack is that it feeds upon itself in the most viscous of circles. The initial wave of panic begins some physiological changes – such as the palpitations and hot flushes etc. which we then feel in turn (and for which there is no obvious cause in our immediate environment), this then intensifies the feeling of anxiety and impending doom, with more physical body changes – and the cycle continues sometimes for a very long time – up to an hour or more in 'waves' – a thoroughly very unpleasant experience, sometimes people pass out – That to me would have been a blessing ! The first method of treatment typically seeks to 'break' the viscous circle as show below:

Panic Attack

Physical Sympoms

E.g. Palpitations, Hot Flush, Clammy skin

Perception & Reaction to Physical Symptoms

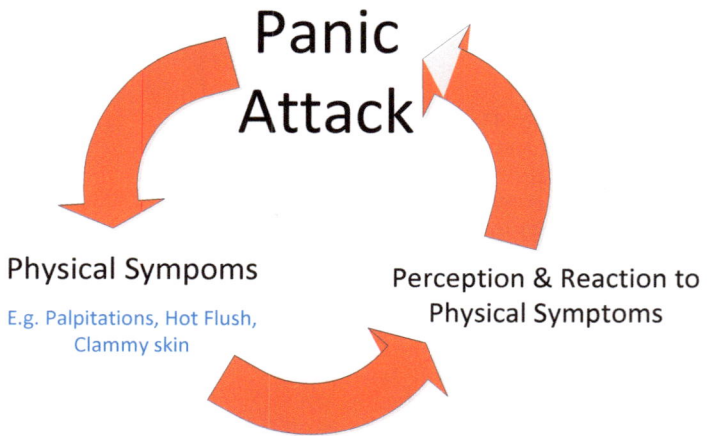

Figure 3 Panic Attack Vicious Circle

So what happens when an individual has a panic disorder or panic attack? An attack begins when a trigger elicits a panic response. This trigger may manifest itself in a variety of ways, from a visual or auditory stimuli, a memory, nightmare or dream (panic disorder may occur in the middle of the night, not to be confused with night terrors). Oftentimes one of the first symptoms is an awareness of rapid heartbeat, or fear of impending doom or even death. Once the individual is aware that their heart rate is racing rapidly, the cycle continues, and actually feeds upon itself. The sympathetic nervous system is triggered, the individual may become diaphoretic (sweaty), and the fight or flight mechanism takes over. At this point, it is very difficult for the individual to stop the cycle.

Breaking the cycle

So how does one break this circle? Basically this is what many treatments seek to do, and many do work in the short term (many don't and it is often a personal thing as to which treatments work the best) – See Treating the Symptoms sections 5 and 7 later.

3. My Panic

First attack

Back in the early 90s my friends and I were basically on a drinking weekend in the south west of Ireland. I was feeling happy as drink could make me and we were camping out on the headland near to the town center. At one point, after enough Guinness, I decided to walk back to the tents; I began not to feel too well. The Irish wind was blowing a gale around me; however the alcohol was acting somewhat as an anesthetic against the cold wind and rain. However half way back, I received what was to be my first panic attack, and to be totally honest its causing me a few problems now describing it. A feeling came over my brain like I'd never ever experienced before and I honestly thought I was getting a brain tumor or something as serious and was about to die. I knew I had been drinking, but I'd never felt like this before with alcohol. It was as if something had 'snapped' in my brain. I retired on my own to my tent, but my brain was still imploding an exploding. I quickly became claustrophobic and had to get out of that tiny tent. Then just as soon as I was out in the open again with the wind howling around my ears, I got intense agoraphobia and had to get back inside the small tent again this back and forth claustrophobia / agoraphobia continued for what seemed like ages. Eventually my friends returned to the tents to find me shivering uncontrollably (I had also probably suffered some exposure). They decided I was in too bad a state to stay camping and moved me to a local B&B for the night. I awoke the next morning to a throbbing head (this time Guinness induced). I sat down to breakfast trying to make sense of the previous night's events, when again the impending doom feeling came over me again, and another panic attack began. I was sure something was desperately wrong with my brain. That was my first and probably most intense panic attack (as I had never before experienced such a feeling). It's one I'll never forget and was probably combined with a dose of exposure.

What caused the Panic Attack?

We can never really know what causes the first attack, although I'm sure the amount of alcohol I drank was definitely a factor, as was a mild case of exposure from the gale on an Irish cliff edge, however probably a major contributing factor was the death of my father a few years earlier, which had affected me badly. There's a well-known psychological theory called 'The safety signal hypothesis' which basically dictates that all of our lives we 'cling on' to certain safety elements in our lives – two of the biggest of which are our parents, who are always there for us, keeping us away from harm and looking after us (see Safety Signal Hypothesis later) When (especially as young adults) we lose one of these safety signals, it can induce intense feelings of anxiety or panic attacks, which are not necessarily immediate in onset. In my case it was a couple of years without my father which apparently induced my first panic attack (helped on by Guinness and an Irish Gale). However everybody's first attack is brought on by their own personal loss or experiences – there is no common pattern, or sometimes obvious cause to the first attack.

Re-Occurrence

My attacks occurred periodically after that following no particular pattern. I would sometimes get one and go out riding on my motorbike to distract myself which probably seems like a crazy thing to do but the driving helped me to concentrate, and I needed to concentrate to try and 'break the cycle'. To be honest in those early days, I really didn't know what was happening or why and I didn't seek professional advice – as I didn't want to admit to myself or anyone else that I might be going crazy. I did take an extended period of leave and travelled for about 9 months which actually did seem to help a lot, however they were always there in the darkest reaches of my brain, hiding and waiting and would soon raise their ugly head again.

When I returned from travelling I went at work at the local university, and for a period of 6 or 7 years had little more trouble with the panic attacks as I was quite content with my personal and career life.

However I did leave the university eventually to get back into private industry, and when I did I encountered a nightmare of a boss. Nothing I could do was good enough for him and every 15 minutes he'd be on the phone asking if I 'd done a particular task yet. I had never encountered a 'boss' like this before, so wasn't really sure what to do, so I just grinned and bared it – I use to almost shake when he was talking to me – it was very unpleasant. – Bad mistake! Unfortunately around this time my other 'safety signal' – my mother died. The panic attacks began again. Eventually I moved Jobs and location to Dublin. There I took another job, which sounded good on paper, but in reality meant I had very little to do, and so was sat for 8 hours a day bored to death – and that really fuelled the panic attacks and anxiety. I again had the 'dread' of going to work in the morning to sit at a desk and do nothing. Eventually I found something better and more active and that really helped my mental health too. I became very involved with the projects I was working on. I also made a major financial commitment by buying myself a house.

After a few years however this job too became boring with little for me to do. I also became committed to a personal relationship and invited my girlfriend to come and live with me. Again the panic attacks began to emerge, this time quite strongly.

At one stage I remember walking to work (about ½ mile) and the anxiety increasing more and more until when I was almost there, I took a full blown panic attack and went down on my honkers on the footpath. I turned around again and went home – and called in sick with 'a headache'. That also brings up the other issue relating to anxiety attacks / panic disorder – it is regarded as a kind of mental illness therefore has a stigma associated with it, and so people (including me at the time) wouldn't admit to having them to your employer. – in case a 'label' stuck. I wonder how many reported stomach aches / or headaches have really been panic attacks.

I would also get them in work – especially as I now was not very busy (bit of a pattern developing here…). Also during meetings – especially in small rooms with lots of people – I'd always try and grab the chair by the door. Trying to stand up and talk and make a meaningful contribution to a meeting whilst in the middle of a full blown panic attack or high anxiety was immensely difficult and I would be nipping myself etc. as a distraction. I wonder how I got through the day sometimes. Sometimes I'd be talking to a work colleague and feel the anxiety begin to increase and I'd have little flinches and lose eye contact with them etc. they probably thought I was being very rude – if only they knew what I was going through. I did tell some work colleagues about them – but never my bosses – I didn't want any kind of sympathy treatment or special case made for me, as it would have been quite embarrassing.

Stimuli of Panic Onset:

At Work

- Long one to one conversations with work colleagues

- Small meeting rooms – especially with overcrowding

- Lack of stimulus / boredom

- Having to 'be' there 8 hours a day at a desk –
  doing nothing!

- Work judgments / assessments – take it to heart
  – judge your whole life by those criteria

At Home

- Watching an emotional scene in a movie / drama

- Hangover

- Work mornings – especially Mondays!

4. What causes Panic Attacks?

There are a number of different theories as to what causes severe anxiety or panic attacks.

Trauma in Childhood

Lipsedge (1993) reported that 58% of patients with agoraphobia had severe disturbances during their upbringing. These included parental illness, violence, and separation. Raskin et al(1982) reported a 70% prevalence of disturbed childhoods in adults with panic disorder.

This may get to the root of your problems, especially if the root of your problems lies in your childhood. Talking to a councilor should help to identify the particular traumas in your own childhood.

Learned Helplessness theory

Martin Seligman (1975) is responsible for the Learned Helplessness theory which had a major influence on psychological research into depression in the 1970s. Seligman discovered helplessness by accident whilst studying the effects of inescapable shock on active avoidance learning in dogs.

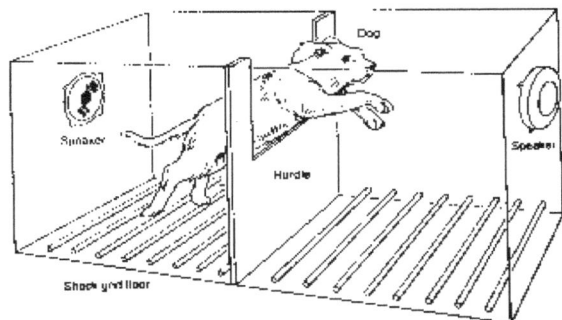

Figure 4 Learned Helplessness Dog Experiment

Seligman restrained dogs in a pavlovian harness and administered several shocks - Unconditioned Stimulus (UCS) paired with a conditioned stimulus (CS) - this is the conventional CS-UCS pairing procedure used to study classical conditioning . Then these dogs were placed in a shuttle-box where they could avoid shock by jumping over a barrier. The shuttle-box was used to study the role of operant conditioning in learning. Most of the dogs failed to learn to avoid shock.

The dogs who were inexperienced with the shock treatment learned fastest to avoid the shocks. The dogs who experienced unavoidable shocks beforehand did not learn and just lay there; they gave up. These experienced dogs lay there and soaked up the shocks because they felt that they had no control over their environment, so they did not try.

Seligman argued that prior exposure to inescapable shock interfered with the ability to learn in a situation where avoidance or escape was possible. Seligman used the term "Learned Helplessness" to describe this phenomenon.

In the late 1970s, Seligman's theory of depression was reformulated within the framework of attribution theory (Gilbert, 1984). Briefly depression will occur if:

- The individual is aware of uncontrollable factors in their environment

- The individual views the situation as unchangeable

They blame themselves for their helplessness – something called "internal attribution".

Safety Signal Hypothesis

The hypothesis that people vividly remember the places in which they have been anxious and associate such locations or situations with symptoms of anxiety, while seeking out situations associated with lowered anxiety.

It is said that humans' basic drive is to control their environment (Stipek, 1988). In turn, if a person has a lack of control over an aspect of their environment in one situation this will impair learning in similar situations. If a person is put in a situation where their behaviour is unaffected, they become passive and their desire to act or try harder dissolves.

To relate this experiment to humans we can look at some individuals who have decided that they have no control over their environment or their lives and so must just lie down and take it – and become depressed, frequently accompanied by panic attacks – due to the perceived 'loss of control'.

Depression

Many people experience sadness following major trauma such as death in the family, divorce or job loss. This is not depression. Depression resembles sadness, but it is more severe and intense. In addition, whereas there is usually a reason for sadness, it can be difficult to account for the severity and intensity of depression in the light of the life events experienced by the sufferer. Indeed 'depression' may be another manifestation of the 'loss of control' mentioned above.

Desensitization

Flying / claustrophobia

If you get panic attacks is claustrophobic situations then one of the best therapies is to frequently expose yourself to as many of these situations as possible (rather than avoid them, which is what your anxiety prompts you to do). Although quite uncomfortable at first (this may be helped by drugs and or relaxation therapy), eventually the level of anxiety will come down, such that you hardly wonder how you ever had this 'irrational' fear over nothing! You basically 'unlearn' the false anxiety response by frequent exposure to the stimulus. One thing is certain if you keep 'avoiding' the anxiety causing stimulus then you will never remove the 'mal-learned 'anxiety response.

5. My Treatment

First Treatment

It was at this point I decided I could take it no more and went to the local doctor. He of course knew about panic attacks and prescribed me some Xanax tranquilizers which were a god send at the time. They really took the edge off them. I kept going back for more, but didn't want to get addicted – but it was of great psychological comfort to know that I always had one in my pocket just in case. My doctor presumed (I don't know why) that I was depressed and also prescribed me anti-depressants (which I didn't take because I wasn't depressed – can you be depressed without knowing it?) and recommend me to a psychologist for counseling. I went gladly, it was the first time in my life I'd ever had to go for counseling, but I didn't care – at this stage I'd try anything.

Counseling

My counselor was foreign (eastern European). She was nice to talk to and I knew she was trying to help, but I could see she was following the textbook treatment methods – relaxation, control your breathing etc. Either this or simply talking about the panic attacks did help to a degree, but there was really no significant improvement. She kept questioning me about my childhood (which by the way was perfect) seeking the root of the problem there – instead of focusing on what was going on in my life right now – which is what she should have focused on. Still it was good to talk to someone about it.

Prescribed drugs

Xanax

This was probably the most effective drug I took it definitely took the edge off the panic attack, however it also had a side-effect of making your thinking a bit hazy. It definitely slowed down your brain – you were definitely not as alert as normal. However as a quick treatment for the panic symptoms I give it 9/10. But it's important not to get psychologically dependent on the drug – use with caution only in a real emergency – and try to reduce the frequency with which you use it for those emergency situations (instead better to have a cognitive coping mechanism) and the amount of drug you use. You can use it very sparingly. I carried a packet of 10 around for a whole year at one stage. You really don't want to cure panic attacks only to find that you've now got a drug dependency! However sometimes just the fact that you **know** you have a quick effective remedy to hand should a panic attack come on is effective enough in lessening the chances of an attack coming on.

Anti-depressants

I have to admit I did try one anti-depressant, out of curiosity, however I found it very strong and didn't like the effect, so I discontinued use. Since then I've noted some have received bad press for inducing suicidal tendencies. However I've known some people who suffer from depression and who swear by anti-depressant drugs, which can take a few weeks to have an effect. However my personal experience was that they weren't very effective against panic attacks. Also I didn't actually feel depressed!

Un Prescribed drugs

Although the fine print on these drugs insist they have natural plant substances to aid anxiety, in reality the main benefit is the placebo effect – whereby you think there's something in the pill that will help, therefore you 'help' yourself mentally (in fact Rescue remedy had quite a high alcohol content – you may as well have a whiskey !). Some of these included:

- St John's Wort

- Calms

- Rescue remedy

My opinion on these 'alternative' remedies is that if they work for you then great. Homeopathy takes this to the extreme by only including minute doses of an ingredient, diluted many times in water. They didn't really work for me as I wasn't convinced there was an 'active' ingredient in any of them. However it's all about 'belief', and if you believe they'll help you then they probably will - to an extent

Relaxation Therapy

In relaxation therapy, you are taught how to relax your body physically and mentally, by lying down, closing your eyes, emptying your thoughts (I was never really sure how to do that!), focusing on a calm scene sometimes accompanied by calming music. You are taught to control your breathing; in fact much of therapy focuses on this. When you feel a high level of anxiety or panic about to occur, you take a deep breath and let the air out slowly, then take another deep one etc. This is combined with tensing your muscles up tight, and then let your shoulders and arm flop down by your sides. I have found that this does help reduce the panic attack symptoms, although it never really 'cured' the panic attack, it's a very quick and easy treatment of the symptoms that you can do pretty much anywhere. You can buy cassette tapes with an expert instructing you in the art of relaxation. Maybe its personal preference, but I preferred a woman's voice – the quality of the voice is also important so try a few different ones. I found this to be the most effective way to 'deal' with a surprise panic attack – take a really deep breath then let it out really slowly. It very effectively demonstrates to yourself that you DO have control.

Music

Music has a huge effect on our mood, and so its potential to relax us cannot be under estimated. There are certain relaxation tapes etc. one can buy with relaxation music, birds singing, waves crashing on the beach (I quite liked that one) as I like being near the coast (despite my first panic attack occurring there !). However musical taste is very much a personal preference, and we all have favourite songs that help us to relax (my personal favourites for this task were Mike Oldfield – Tubular Bells, and Rainbow Live on Stage – Catch the Rainbow – both a whole (LP) side long, so at least 20mins of music to calm me down). It's a good idea to make a tape or CD with a collection of your favourite calming tunes which you can just put on whenever you need to calm down. If need be carry a tape / CD / mp3 player wherever you go. If can play an instrument, this is also a useful way to engage in calming down, I would sometimes play guitar – not any particular tune, just a sequence of chords over and over again and vary the rhythm faster and slower and found that this helped me to focus and calm myself.

Exercise

Exercise is another good way to release tension and relax – although it's not always appropriate to the context/environment (e.g. work office) that you're in. It's difficult for the fight or flight adrenaline to create a panic attack when it's all been used up in a bout of exercise! I personally found a good game of squash really helped me to forget the outside world, any troubles I had (including anxiety/panic attacks). For 45 minutes I emptied my head of everything except 4 white walls and a little black ball. You have to react so quickly in a game of squash that you don't have time to think about anything else – including panic attacks.

Hypnotherapy

Expert Hypnosis

I got to the stage that I decided to give hypnosis a go – even though I could barely afford it, I booked myself in for 8 sessions with a renowned hypnotist. As part of the therapy they gave me a series of tapes which I was supposed to listed to a couple of hours each day – which I did on the way to work and back again. The tapes basically had the chief hypnotist conducting relaxation and positive thinking exercises with you. Some of it sounded a bit silly to be honest, but I played along, as I was determined. In the hypnosis sessions, I was led into a small room with pastel colours, a warm glow and some relaxing music playing softly in the background. Here they would leave you for 10 minutes to relax yourself, then a therapist would come in and basically conduct relaxation therapy with you. After about the 4th session I was left lying in the room with my eyes closed, when another person entered the room – it was the voice from the tapes which I had supposedly been 'conditioned' to. The voice told me to close my eyes and imaging there were weights on them and that I wouldn't be able to open them. Eventually the voice instructed me to try to open my eyes – which I did and looked straight at him – to his disappointment (and mine!). I guess I just couldn't be hypnotized (some people can't), even though I wanted to be, or maybe I was at such a level of anxiety that I couldn't slip into that hypnotic state of mind. I did find the sessions relaxing; however I was never hypnotized and felt It was bit of a waste of money, but I had to try – it does work for some people! It may work for you – it's definitely worth a try!

Self-Hypnosis

Another form of hypnosis which I hadn't heard of before is self-hypnosis, which to me sounded like a contradiction in terms – how can you hypnotize yourself ? If you did how would you snap out of it ? However the truth is that we all do this occasionally – usually when we're in quite a relaxed mood, perhaps just sitting waiting in a queue, or on a bus, looking out of a window, staring at that dot on the ceiling, your mind just drifts and kind of empties, or thinks about far off people and places. It may only be for a few seconds or several minutes, but eventually you are brought back to the present usually by someone saying "Where did you go off to ?" or an abrupt noise. Next time you do this try and realize that it is actually a form of self-hypnosis, so that you can use it again in times of high anxiety. However personally I found it very difficult to return to that 'drift away' state from a heightened state of anxiety.

Cognitive Therapy

There exist a number of different 'cognitive' therapies which purport to changing your way of thinking – they include positive thinking and focusing on longer term goals going to 'your happy place' etc. Which are fine when you're feeling fine, but in the context of a full blown panic attack are extremely difficult to do. Instead I have to say that erotic thoughts (and I'll not go into any more detail than that!) came much easier and were much more useful as a 'cognitive distraction' therapy. My theory is that if your basic instincts (fight/flight anxiety) are working against you, then fight them with another basic instinct – the sex drive! Probably not recommend by the doctors, but it worked for me☺.

6. Stressors

The key in my view to panic attacks is identifying and removing (or reducing) the stressors in your life – the things that are pulling at you from different directions (see Figure 5).

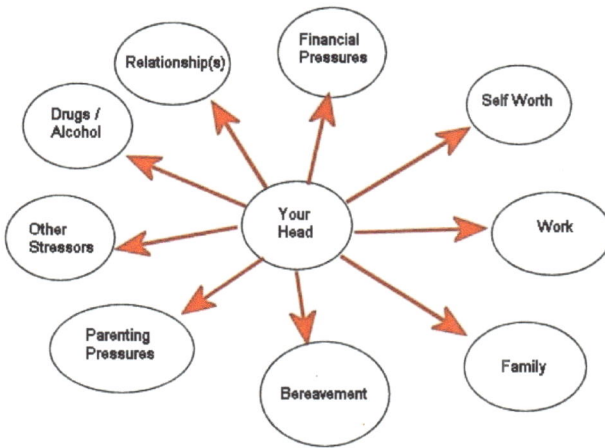

Figure 5 Potential Stressors Pulling at your life

I'm pretty sure that although my initial panic attacks were brought on by delayed paternal grief and loss of 'safety' signal. However whenever a series of different stressors began to build up all around me, something had to give – and eventually it did – my brain resorted to that earlier anxious state that belatedly accompanied my parents deaths and went into panic attack mode to let me know that things were not good !

Identify your Stressors!

The main problem is identifying the stressors (and admitting that they are stressors).They may be financial, relationship, work related, self-worth related etc. or combinations of all of these and more. You have to ask yourself has there been a sudden change in your life's circumstances or even a gradual one that has finally reached an unacceptable limit.

What has changed in your life recently?

- Job

- Financial pressure

- Overwork

- Relationship Status

- Under work / Under Stimulation

Self-Worth

Have you recently failed an exam or course or over a period of time developed negative thoughts about your own perceived worth amongst your family, peers, work colleagues or society in general.

Relationship(s)

Are you currently in an abusive or 'difficult relationship that you can't see a way out of (e.g. due to family commitments housing arrangements or childcare commitments)?

Financial

Have you recently taken on a large financial burden (e.g. mortgage/ loan) or invested or over-spent your budget and things have gotten out of hand?

Overwork / Underwork

Have you recently taken on more at work than you can handle and can't cope with the pressure and deadlines? Have you been given less to do and are thoroughly bored?

Drugs / Alcohol

Have you recently developed a dependency on drugs or alcohol with knock-on consequences to your job / relationship or health? Are you now over-indulging in order to 'cope' with the panic attacks?

Binge drinking

Panic disorder can coexist with other illnesses such as depression and substance abuse. Approximately 30-45% of individuals with panic disorder do go on to abuse alcohol. This makes total clinical sense since they are trying to self-medicate to decrease the panic disorder they are having. Around 20% do above other substances. Marijuana is a typically abused substance for these individuals. Some abuse cocaine, although a few studies have shown that panic disorder may be elicited in individuals who frequently abuse cocaine. It is very unusual for a pre-existing panic disorder patient to begin abusing cocaine, as symptoms similar to panic disorder may result.

Parenting Demands

Have you recently become a parent? It is all a bit overwhelming? Do you perceive conflicting demands from your child / their siblings / the Education system / your own career / health issues etc.?

Interaction of stressors – multi-stressor effect

It could be the case that a single stressor may not be responsible for your panic attacks / anxiety. Instead there may be an interaction of a number of minor stressors which ends up resulting in a major stressor effect which develops into a 'loss of control' and potential panic attacks or anxiety.

7. Treat the Stressors

Once you treat the stressors then you're focussing on the 'causes' of your panic attacks rather than just the symptoms. It is important to treat the symptoms e.g. with short term use of anti-anxiety drugs or relaxation and breathing exercises, but ultimately you need to treat the 'disease' rather than the symptoms. The 'disease' in this case is the stressors in your life.

Remove the Stressor

Ideally this should be your goal, however it is not always immediately possible – which is part of the reason why it's a stressor in the first place. If you can't immediately remove it then think about ways to cope with it that will cause you less stress. You may need to make sacrifices or trade-offs in order to 'deal' with a stressor. In addition you should make a plan on how to remove the stressor completely. Write down the plan; break it down into mini-steps that are achievable even in the short term. It's important to achieve mini-steps in order to see yourself making progress towards ultimately removing the stressor from your life.

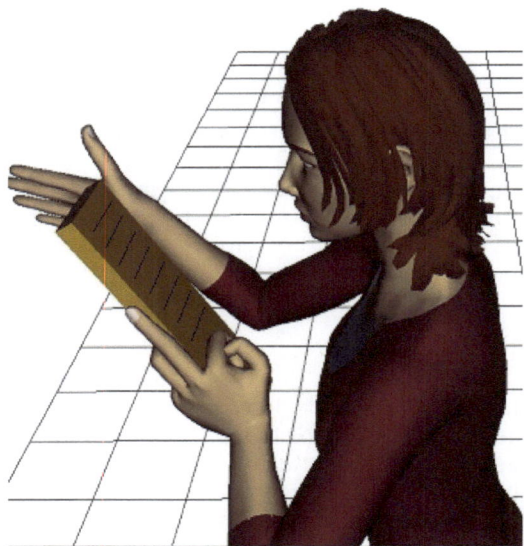

Figure 6 Make a plan and break it down into steps

Resolve the Stressor

If you can't immediately remove the stressor then try and resolve it either directly or through an intermediary. This could mean sitting down to write a letter / email or making a phone call or sitting down to talk to relevant people or just friends who are there to help you out. Resolving the issue / stressor may (as in remove above) involve making sacrifices and or trade-offs which in turn may create more stressors – thus a vicious circle can begin, however it may have less stressful effects on you and thus may be worth making the sacrifice to alleviate your mental health !

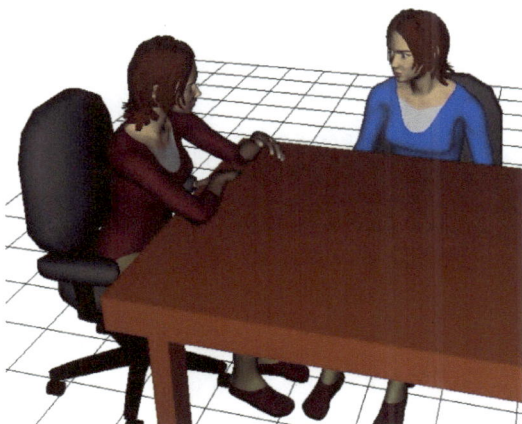

Figure 7 Talk it over with a friend

Stimulate your brain

Distraction is a good way to move your brain on from thinking negative thoughts and focusing on the stressors in your life. It might be an idea to learn a new skill e.g. computer skills or take up a creative hobby like painting or model making or gardening. Consider getting a pet – looking after another's needs is a good distractor from your own. It's also relaxing! If your stressor involves under-work or boredom e.g. at your job, then use the time to try and learn a new skill or be creative and write a book or create some art or tools that could help you whenever you eventually do get busy again.

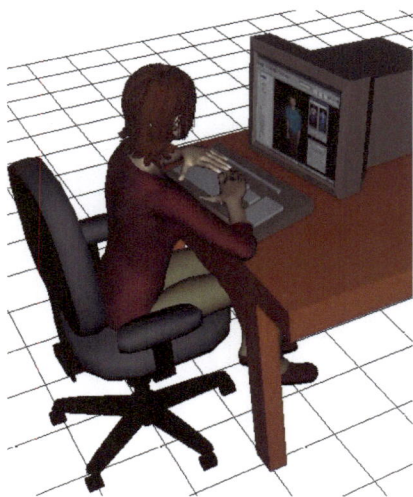

Figure 8 Stimulate your brain

Regain Control

Try and regain some control of the stressors or elements relating to them. If you can show to yourself that you have at least some degree of control over your stressors then you'll be taking big steps in relieving the causes of the panic attacks.

It may require some big life changes as you may have 'drifted' into the current situation by not taking action / steps to avoid it for quite a long time. For example it could mean quitting your job (which would have major financial consequences) or ending a bad or damaged relationship (which could also have financial and / or emotional consequences).

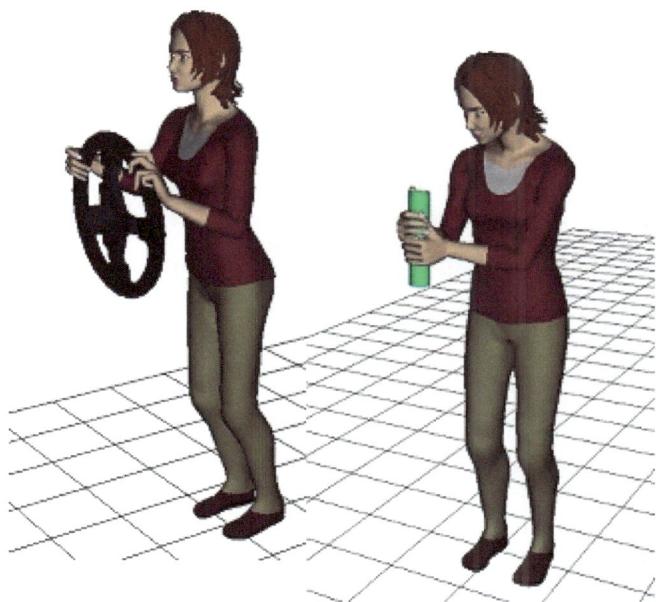

Figure 9 Take back Control

Setting Life Goals

- Life goal over-rides career goal

- What makes you happy

- What do you like doing ? Try work at that

- me: Creative / music / graphics / writing / photography

- What did you like as a child

- What makes you laugh

8. Conclusion

In conclusion I can say that there are no quick fixes. There *are* quick fixes for the *symptoms* (i.e. the panic attack itself), such as relaxation breathing exercises and anti-anxiety drugs (or just having the drugs at hand). It's good to have these as an 'emergency' coping strategy. However the underlying *causes* (the stressors) require some degree of self-analysis, an action plan on how to resolve and / or remove those stressors and then implementation of that plan, even if its only baby steps at first. It maybe that you need help to address these so don't be afraid to ask for it. You may also have to make trade-offs or compromises and incur the consequences of those. However if they will result in less stress than you're currently enduring then surely its worth making these compromises.

If you really want to 'cure' yourself of the panic attacks then you have to:

- Have the courage to make change

- Set real goals – with real steps

Am I cured?

Am I cured? I'd say 90%, but the ugly beast could arise again at any point (now that I know I'm susceptible to it). The long term solution is really remove those stressors take control, identify what you like – make steps to achieve it and go get it. DON'T suffer a job or relationship problem etc. in silence – do something about it – the sooner the better. And lastly try to be optimistic, life is fun – smile more and people will smile back really – try it ☺.

"I am no longer accepting the things I cannot change

It is time to change the things I cannot accept"

Angela Davis

9. References

Gilbert, Depression: From Psychology to Brain State, Lawrence. Erlbaum Associates, London, 1984.

Lipsedge MS, Chapter 14, in Bowlby J: Separation. New York, Basic Books, 1993.

Raskin M, Peeke HV, Dickman W, et al: Panic and generalized anxiety disorders: Developmental antecedents and precipitants. Arch Gen Psychiatry 39:687-689, 1982.

Seligman, Martin E. P. (1975). Learned helplessness: Depression, development and death. W. H. Freeman: New York Stipek, D. E. P. (1988). Motivation to learning. Allyn & Bacon: Boston.

www.ingramcontent.com/pod-product-compliance
Lightning Source LLC
Chambersburg PA
CBHW041718200326
41520CB00001B/150